Drug Abuse and Society™

PRESCRIPTION DRUGS

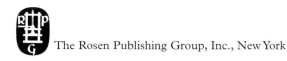

The Rosen Publishing Group, Inc., New York

Fred Ramen

For Dr. Kate

Published in 2007 by The Rosen Publishing Group, Inc.
29 East 21st Street, New York, NY 10010

Library of Congress Cataloging-in-Publication Data

Ramen, Fred.
Prescription drugs / Fred Ramen.—1st ed.
   p. cm.—(Drug abuse and society)
Includes bibliographical references and index.
ISBN-13: 978-1-4042-0915-2
ISBN-10: 1-4042-0915-8 (library binding)
1. Medication abuse. 2. Drugs.
I. Title. II. Series.
RM146.5R36 2007
615'.1—dc22

2006009409

Manufactured in the United States of America

Contents

Introduction   **4**

CHAPTER 1 The History and Physiology of Prescription Drug Abuse   **8**

CHAPTER 2 Use and Abuse   **17**

CHAPTER 3 Coping with Abuse   **23**

CHAPTER 4 Prescription Drugs and the Legal System   **32**

CHAPTER 5 Prescription Drug Abuse and Society   **40**

CHAPTER 6 Prescription Drug Abuse and the Media   **46**

Glossary   **54**

For More Information   **57**

For Further Reading   **59**

Bibliography   **61**

Index   **62**

INTRODUCTION

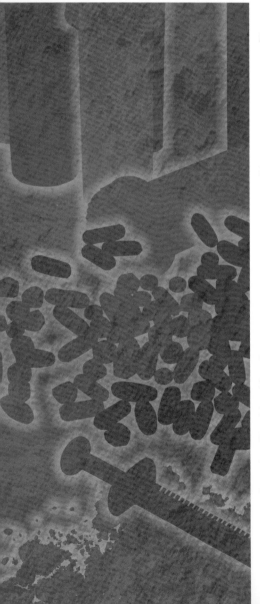

"Out of ten people I know, maybe one has seen or tried cocaine, but nine of them have done Ritalin."
—High school student, Bethesda, Maryland

"It was a very gradual thing. It never occurred to me that I had a drug problem."
—Justin, attorney and former prescription drug abuser

When most people think of drug abuse, they think of the many street drugs—such as heroin, cocaine, marijuana, and ecstasy—that are familiar to them from newspapers, movies, and television. They would be surprised, however, to know that almost three million Americans a year abuse drugs that most people assume are safe,

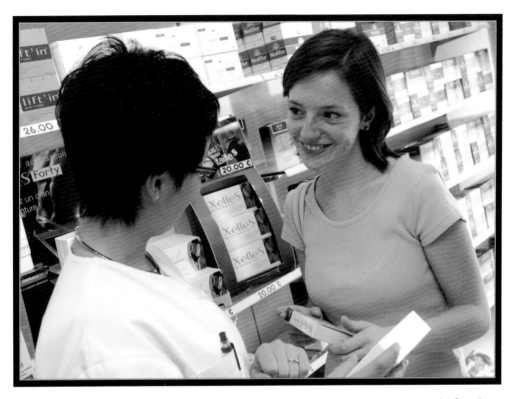

Every day, millions of Americans, including many teenagers, quietly feed their drug addictions at the local pharmacy. This hidden epidemic is one of America's greatest health-care challenges.

were often prescribed by a physician, and were bought at the corner pharmacy.

An alarming trend is the rise in the abuse of these prescription drugs among young people. A 2005 study by the Partnership for a Drug-Free America revealed that one in ten teenagers has used prescription medication to get high, and one in ten has abused over-the-counter (OTC) drugs such as cough syrup. This means that teens are more likely to abuse prescription drugs than illegal drugs, like cocaine and GHB (gamma hydroxybutyrate).

Prescription drug abuse may be hard to detect for both an addict and his or her friends and family. Because the drugs initially come from a doctor, many people assume that they are safe or not addictive. Because they most often get their drugs from a legal drugstore, abusers may not even think of themselves as addicts. But their addiction is real and often has a devastating effect on their lives and families.

This book will examine the different kinds of prescription drugs that are commonly abused. These include stimulants such as Ritalin and Adderall, tranquilizers such as Xanax, and painkillers such as codeine and Demerol. We will learn how these drugs work in the body, why they are prescribed, and why some people develop a dangerous addiction to them. We will also look at the consequences of abuse on people, from the physical effects of the drugs themselves to the terrible toll they inflict on the people around them.

We will also examine the many ways that addiction can be treated. Although it is a long and difficult road, there is a way out for every addict. However, addiction is not something that can be overcome simply by a desire to quit, even though the addict must first want to stop taking the drug. Addictive drugs change the abuser's body and even alter the structure of the brain. Although many people withdraw on their own, direct medical supervision is the safest and most supportive way to withdraw from an addictive substance.

We will also look at the ways that people are able to get prescription drugs and identify some of the warning signs of addiction. Although these drugs are prescribed by a physician, abusing them is a crime. Therefore, we will examine the legal consequences of supporting such a drug habit. Finally, we will explore how the media have portrayed the problem of prescription drug abuse, which remains an underreported problem.

CHAPTER 1

The History and Physiology of Prescription Drug Abuse

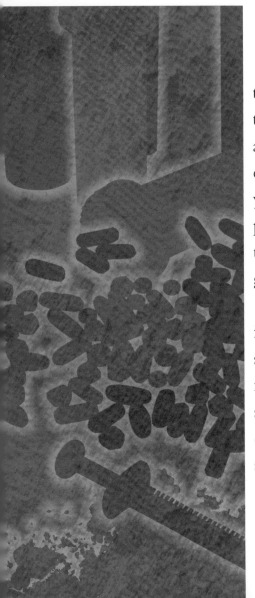

For as long as physicians and healers have been prescribing remedies to their patients, people have abused these substances, using them to make themselves feel better beyond treating an ailment. With the advances in medical science that have occurred in the last 200 years, people now have access to more powerful drugs than ever before. As a result, the abuse of these drugs has become a bigger problem.

Any drug can be dangerous if used incorrectly. Because prescription drugs are so powerful, they can be very dangerous indeed. The most frequently abused prescription drugs fall into three basic categories: painkillers, tranquilizers, and stimulants.

PAINKILLERS

As the name indicates, a painkiller is a medicine that is used to relieve pain. Some of the most powerful painkillers are opioids. These drugs are descendants of opium, a powerful narcotic made from the opium poppy that makes users very drowsy, insensitive to pain, and prone to hallucinations. Opioids were originally

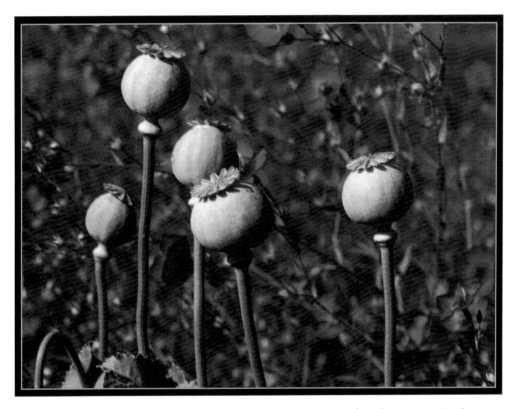

Papaver somniferum, the opium poppy, is the source for the narcotic drug opium and its derivative, heroin. While many useful painkillers can be made from the opium poppy, all of them carry the risk of addiction.

manufactured directly from opium. Today's more powerful opioids are created in laboratories from various chemicals.

Opioids are extremely potent and are, therefore, quite addictive. The most famous illegal opioid is heroin, which is most often injected or snorted by its users. A weaker version of heroin is morphine, which has been used as a painkiller since the eighteenth century. One of the first widespread drug problems in the United States was the addiction to morphine among wounded veterans of the Civil War. Doctors of that time did not realize how addictive the drug could be and often overprescribed it when treating soldiers.

Other commonly prescribed opioids are codeine (often given for mild to moderate pain), Vicodin (for more severe pain, especially back or joint injuries), Demerol, and oxycodone (OxyContin). Although these drugs are safe if they're taken according to a doctor's instructions, the potential for abuse is very real. This is especially true if the patient has had a prior problem with addiction, either to another drug or to alcohol.

Opioids work by attaching to receptor sites on the nerves in the brain, spinal cord, and internal organs. When an opioid attaches to these receptors, the nerves no longer respond to pain impulses. The drug can also produce a feeling of happiness or euphoria. Because of this, people often begin to abuse the drug in search of the euphoric sensation. However, the body quickly becomes accustomed to the opioid, and the user needs to take more and

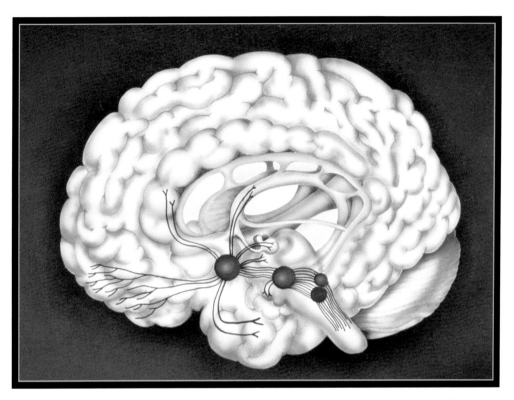

This diagram of the brain shows the parts affected by opioid drugs. Opioids affect the function of many important regions of the brain. This includes the brain stem, which regulates many bodily functions, and the hypothalamus and thalamus, which regulate the endocrine system and sensory inputs to the brain.

more of it to get high. This condition is called tolerance. Worse, the body also begins to crave the drug, and the user needs to take it to not feel sick. This is called dependency, and it is one of the reasons opioid addiction is so hard to treat. When a person does not get the drug, he or she begins to feel very sick and go through withdrawal symptoms. Opioid withdrawal usually causes intense muscle pain, shaking, nausea, depression, and cold flashes.

TRANQUILIZERS

Tranquilizers are drugs that depress, or slow, the functioning of the nervous system and brain. Because of this, they are often called central nervous system (CNS) depressants. CNS depressants are used to treat nervousness, anxiety, and insomnia.

There are two main categories of CNS depressants: barbiturates and benzodiazepines. Barbiturates are the older type of this class of drug. They are very effective at sedating (making sleepy) the person who uses them, but they can be very dangerous as well. Barbiturate overdoses are often deadly, and the user must be very careful about consuming alcohol while using the drugs, as that can increase the chances of an overdose.

Benzodiazepines are a newer class of tranquilizers. The first commonly prescribed benzodiazepine was Valium (diazepam), which appeared in 1963. At first, it was thought that these drugs were very safe, but within ten years doctors realized that it was possible to become addicted to them. Modern benzodiazepines include Xanax (alprazolam) and Halcion (triazolam). They are usually prescribed only for short-term periods or for occasional, not daily, use.

Withdrawal from CNS depressants can be difficult. Although benzodiazepines are generally safer than barbiturates to take and stop taking, getting off them must be done under the supervision of medical personnel. To abruptly stop taking the drug—going "cold turkey"—can cause seizures and other medical problems, which can be life-threatening. Even when taking these drugs properly, it is important to gradually reduce the dosage so that the body can slowly become accustomed to doing without them.

MYTHS AND FACTS

Myth: Prescription drugs are always safe.

Fact: Like all drugs, prescription drugs can be dangerous if taken without a doctor's supervision. Even drugs sold over the counter (OTC) can be deadly if you take too many or take them with other drugs. Always discuss the drugs you are taking with a doctor when he or she wants to prescribe a new treatment for you.

Myth: Prescription drugs are not addictive.

Fact: Many prescription drugs can be quite addictive. Never take more of any drug than your doctor recommends, and never take drugs that were not prescribed for you.

Myth: You can stop taking prescription drugs whenever you want to.

Fact: Many drugs that doctors prescribe build up in your body over time. Quitting suddenly can cause your body to go into shock as it is deprived of the drugs. Always follow doctors' instructions for ending a prescription.

13

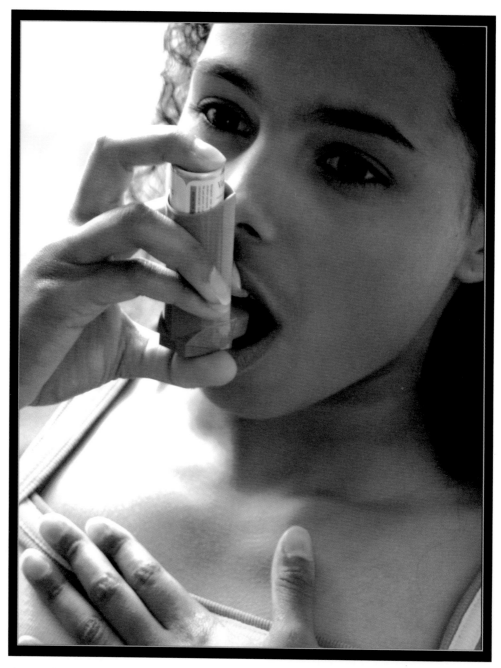

An asthma patient uses an inhaler. Inhalers contain powerful stimulants that help open the constricted passageways in the lungs. Prescription drug abusers sometimes use inhalers for the high these stimulants can cause in people not suffering an asthma attack.

Usually, you will have to take smaller and smaller doses until your body is used to not having the drug anymore.

STIMULANTS

Unlike CNS depressants, stimulants increase the functioning of the nervous system. They also raise heart and respiration rates. Illegal stimulants include Benzedrine (speed), methamphetamine (crystal meth), and cocaine. Stimulants were once recommended for asthma sufferers (they help to force open the constricted breathing passages of a person having an asthma attack) and for dieters (because they raise a person's metabolism—the rate energy is burned—and suppress the appetite). However, stimulants can be very addictive. They can produce a powerful high and a feeling of invincibility (the ability to do anything). Stimulants also interfere with the user's ability to make decisions. Once the high wears off, a user often becomes depressed and begins to abuse the drug to feel better again. Because of this, stimulants are prescribed less today, and only for a few conditions such as narcolepsy and ADHD.

One area in which the use of stimulants has grown, however, is in the treatment of attention deficit hyperactivity disorder (ADHD). People with this disorder often have problems concentrating, paying attention to ordinary tasks, and focusing in general. Doctors use the stimulant Ritalin (methylphenidate) to treat ADHD. Those who support its use claim that, in small doses, Ritalin seems to improve the ability of a person to concentrate and actually calms him or her down—despite the fact that stimulants generally cause people to become more active.

Ritalin use has become more controversial as doctors have increasingly prescribed it. Moreover, there is strong evidence that it is being abused, often by people for whom the drug was not prescribed.

The use of stimulants can be risky. Repeated abuse can lead to feelings of paranoia and rage, as well as damage to the cardio-vascular system. Stimulants can also cause a person to develop a dangerously high fever, or even go into seizures.

CHAPTER 2

Use and Abuse

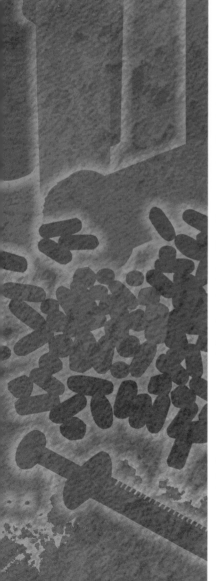

No one sets out to become a drug addict. What's unique about prescription drug abusers is that most of them first encounter the substances legally. Because of this, the descent into addiction can go untreated much longer than it would with illegal drugs.

Most people who are prescribed powerful drugs never abuse them or develop an addiction to them. By far, the majority of people take them for a while and then stop using them. However, some begin to abuse the drugs and, if not caught in time, may become addicted to them.

WHO'S AT RISK

Anyone can become addicted to a drug. However, there are warning factors that

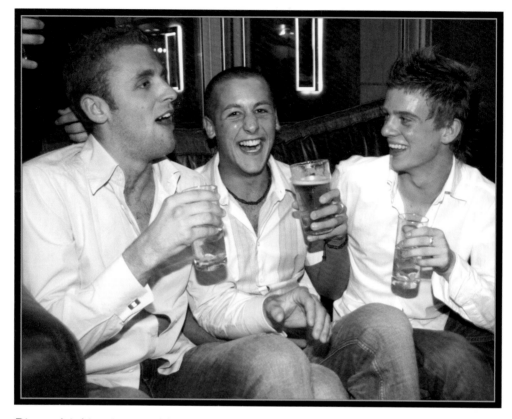

Binge drinking is a problem among many young people, especially college students away from home for the first time. People who have abused alcohol are at a higher risk of developing a prescription drug problem.

indicate a person may be more likely to develop a drug abuse problem. People who have physical conditions that require pain medication, like joint or back injuries or chronic diseases, need to be carefully monitored if they are prescribed other drugs such as benzodiazepines. Likewise, people who drink heavily may already have an addiction to alcohol and are therefore at a greater risk of developing other substance abuse problems.

Fatigue, stress, depression, and obesity are other risk factors that make a person more likely to abuse drugs.

More women than men become addicted to prescription drugs, probably because they are two to three times more likely than men to be prescribed drugs such as tranquilizers. In addition, the user's age can influence the likelihood of his or her abusing drugs. Seniors and teenagers are more likely to abuse drugs than people in other age groups. Why? Seniors are more likely to be prescribed powerful drugs, and adolescents are at a vulnerable period in their life and may begin to abuse drugs without fully understanding the consequences of their actions.

GETTING THE DRUGS

A person who becomes addicted to any drug has many challenges. The first challenge is the need to secure a large supply. Addicts need greater doses of the drug they are addicted to. In the case of prescription drug abusers, this can be as high as twenty or thirty times the normal dose. Recovering addicts often recall that the first thing on their minds when they woke up was how to get enough drugs to last the day. Without enough, they will go into withdrawal and suffer its terrible symptoms. Even worse, most started to take the prescription drug to help them with a problem, like pain or emotional distress. Because their bodies have built up such a tolerance to the drug, however, they need larger doses to feel the effects. Without the drugs, the original symptoms will return, making life doubly difficult for addicts.

Addicts do not usually have to turn to drug dealers to get their supply, although many dealers do sell prescription drugs. Instead, addicts turn to clean, safe pharmacies for their supply. All they need is a prescription, and they can get as much as they want.

Getting a prescription can be difficult, however. Most addictive prescription drugs are carefully controlled and monitored. Doctors have to carefully note how often they prescribe these drugs to patients—not only for the health of the patient, but also to make sure they do not become, in effect, drug dealers.

Many prescription drug addicts go "doctor shopping." This means they go to several different doctors so that their pattern of abuse goes unnoticed. They also look for doctors who will turn a blind eye to their abuse.

Emergency rooms are a good source of prescriptions, partly because the doctors there are often too busy to follow up with patients who come in. Moreover, it is easier for patients to use fake names in emergency rooms.

As a last resort, some addicts steal or try to forge the prescription pads doctors use, so that they can write as many prescriptions as they want.

Even when a prescription is secured, addicts must be careful about where they fill it. Pharmacies keep track of how often they can fill a prescription, for insurance purposes and to catch

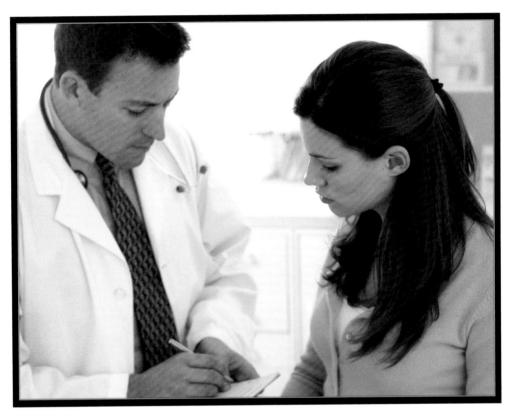

Doctors write their prescriptions on special pads. These prescription pads are designed to be difficult to photocopy, to prevent people from improperly obtaining drugs. Prescription drug addicts often try to steal these pads in order to get the drug they are addicted to.

people who are trying to get large amounts of drugs. Addicts typically visit many different pharmacies, being careful not to drop by any one too often.

Sadly, health-care workers are sometimes abusers themselves or are willing sources for illegally acquired prescription drugs. Doctors and nurses face enormous pressure on their jobs, and many begin to self-medicate, perhaps believing that they will be

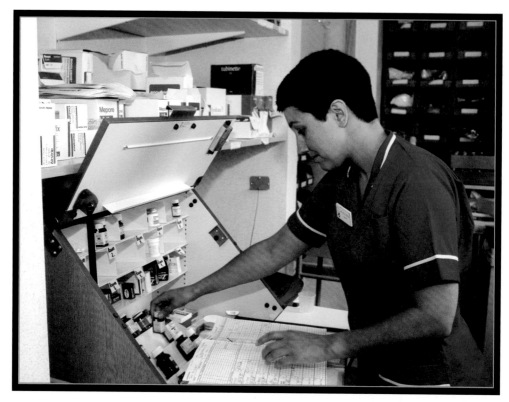

Hospitals need to maintain control over the powerful drugs they keep on hand. Here, a nurse is checking the drugs for each patient she is responsible for. Note that she must keep careful track of how much of each drug she uses, and how much is left.

able to control their use. Although there are tight controls on addictive drugs, it is possible to circumvent them for a time, and health-care workers have frequent access to these drugs. Inevitably, these users are caught, often with devastating consequences to their lives and careers.

CHAPTER 3

Coping with Abuse

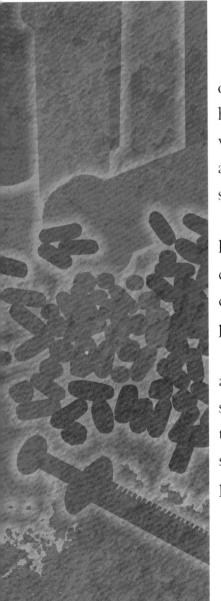

Michelle was an active teenager who enjoyed spending time with her friends and being a member of her school's cheerleading squad. During her senior year, Michelle went on a ski trip with some classmates. While going down a tricky slope, she fell hard and hit a tree, shattering her left leg.

Doctors had to perform surgery to set her leg, and afterwards she was in a great deal of pain. To help her get through the day, doctors prescribed Vicodin, an opioid painkiller.

Michelle had been known to get drunk at parties before, although nobody thought she had a problem with alcohol. However, that may have been the first warning sign that she might become addicted to painkillers.

At first, Michelle only took the Vicodin as directed. Then she began to go beyond the prescribed dosage, often taking two or more of the pills at the same time. Vicodin did more than just take away her pain—it made her feel good. Perhaps that is why she began to take more of it than she needed.

Michelle discovered she needed to take higher doses just to make the pain go away. She got worried, and one weekend she tried not to take Vicodin at all. It was terrible: she felt sick to her stomach, got chills, and shook uncontrollably. Finally, she broke down and took some pills, which made her feel better. The experience terrified her and she never wanted to go through it again.

Gradually, Michelle began to lose interest in anything but finding more Vicodin. Although she had finished her rehabilitation, she quit the cheerleading squad. She broke up with her boyfriend. She started hanging around with a different group of friends. Many of them were drug users, and they helped her to find pills.

Michelle's quest for medication became a major part of her everyday life. Her doctor would only write a prescription for a small amount of what she wanted. She began to go to different emergency rooms in her town, faking symptoms to get a prescription for painkillers. By now, Michelle was familiar with many different kinds—Demerol, MS Contin, and Percocet—and she knew exactly what to tell doctors to fool them into prescribing them to her.

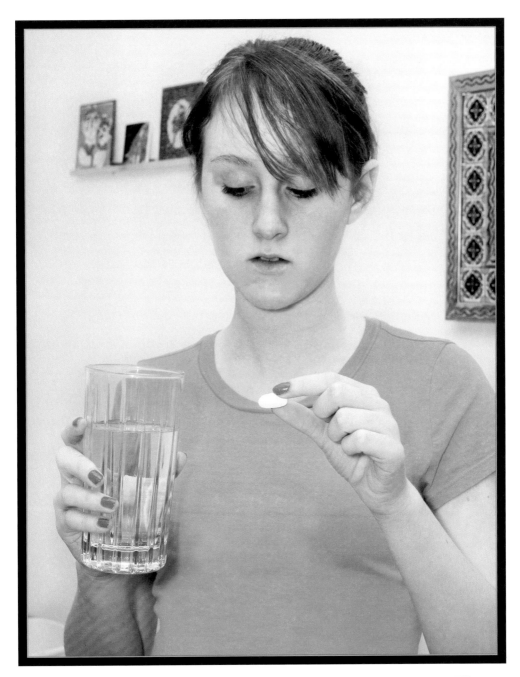

Life often quickly becomes a struggle for prescription drug addicts. They wake up every morning worrying about how to find enough pills to get them through the day. Getting pills often means more to them than anything else, including friends and family.

Even when Michelle could get a prescription, the drugs were still very expensive. She quickly used up all the money she had saved from her allowance and the job she had over the summer. She began to steal from her parents, taking cash from where they kept it in their bedroom. Her parents noticed the money was missing and stopped putting it there. Michelle then began to sell some of her mother's jewelry. She found her parents' credit card numbers and used them to buy things such as television and clothes that she could sell quickly. Eventually, she maxed out the cards and her parents found out.

By now, Michelle barely went to school at all. She spent most of her time with other drug addicts. Sometimes, they broke into houses and stole things to help pay for their habit. Her parents finally confronted her about her drug problem and begged her to let them get help for her. In response, Michelle ran away from home and went to a large city nearby.

For a time, she was able to survive by working low-paying jobs for a few days, until she made enough money to buy more pills. She was taking almost thirty a day now, and every day was a struggle to find more. On one visit to a hospital, though, Michelle managed to steal a prescription pad from the doctor. She now could get all the drugs she craved. She thought her problems were over, but in actuality this was just the last step before she bottomed out.

Although she tried to be careful about where she got her prescription filled, the drugs made her confused. One day, she made the mistake of going to the same pharmacy twice. The pharmacist called the doctor on the prescription to confirm the order. When he found out it had been forged, he called the police. Michelle was arrested when she returned to pick up the prescription.

She was terrified of jail. She called her parents, and they bailed her out on the condition that she seek treatment. She moved back home with them and started to participate in a drug treatment program. Eventually, Michelle had to go to a clinic, where she was taken off the drugs. It took several weeks, during which she suffered from severe withdrawal symptoms, but she became clean. She entered Narcotics Anonymous, a twelve-step program for former addicts, and started taking classes to get her high school diploma.

Today, Michelle is attending a community college. She also works as a drug counselor for her local treatment program. She shares her experiences so that she can help others overcome their addictions before they hit bottom like she did.

OVERCOMING ADDICTION

Nobody knows for certain why some people become addicted to drugs. Scientists believe there are many possible causes. Heredity seems to play a part, but there may be many different genes that can make a person susceptible to drug abuse. There are also psychological factors involved. For example, people who are depressed are at a greater risk. In the story above, Michelle's

Misuse, Abuse, and Addiction

People in the health-care community use three different terms—misuse, abuse, and addiction—to describe the ways people use prescription drugs improperly.

"Misuse" means taking a drug incorrectly. If you use a prescription drug that was not given to you by a doctor, you are misusing the drug, just as you are if you stop taking a drug that was prescribed to you before you are supposed to. Using prescription drugs and alcohol together is also misuse in many cases. Some studies have shown that up to 50 percent of all prescriptions are not used correctly, leading to more than 200,000 deaths a year.

"Abuse" means using a drug for reasons not related to its intended purpose, such as taking it to get high or taking more of it than you were prescribed. Abuse may or may not lead to addiction, but it is dangerous.

"Addiction" (or dependency) means that a person is always craving the drug and needs it to feel "normal." Addicts will place getting the drug they are hooked on above all other concerns, even food. Their bodies have become dependent on the drug, and they must have it to avoid withdrawal. Addiction will continue to get worse if it is not treated. Very often, the addiction will be fatal, no matter what drug the user is taking.

occasional overuse of alcohol was perhaps a signal that she might be at risk for developing a drug problem. However, it certainly wasn't a definite sign that she would become an addict.

The most important step in recovery is for the addict to want to stop being dependent on the drug. For many, this only happens when they have hit bottom. In other words, they have had so many bad things happen to them because of their addiction that they can't live with themselves anymore. Often, hitting bottom occurs when they are arrested, as was the case with Michelle. Drug counselors, many of whom are former addicts themselves, try to educate people with substance-abuse problems so that they will seek help before they reach their lowest points.

THE DIFFICULTIES OF RECOVERY

There are two problems to overcome when a person wants to recover from being an addict. The first is to end the physical dependence on the drug, a process called detoxification, or detox. The drug must be completely out of the user's system. Detoxification involves going through withdrawal, which is why this part of recovery is best done in a medical setting. Doctors will usually help the patient by giving him or her smaller and smaller doses of the drug to wean the body from its dependence. Even so, the physical symptoms of withdrawal will probably occur at some point, and these can be intense and debilitating.

Some of the most difficult drugs to stop using are the benzodiazepines. These have very long half-lives (the period of time it takes for the amount of drugs in the body to be reduced in half), and the body itself becomes very dependent upon these drugs. While some users of illicit drugs or alcohol can detox in as little as three days, it can take up to two weeks for users of benzodiazepines to fully detox.

On the other hand, some users of opioid drugs opt for a process called rapid detox. These patients are put under general anesthesia, making them unconscious, and then a drug that destroys the opioids in their systems is injected. Over a six-hour period, the users go through withdrawal but remain unconscious the whole time. When they wake up, they have been fully detoxified. This procedure seems effective but remains controversial because it uses general anesthesia, which always carries a risk of death or brain damage.

The second problem is the psychological dependence on the drug. For a long time, the addiction to the drug created stress in the addict's life, stress that he or she dealt with by taking drugs. The addict must now learn how to cope with stress without taking the drug. Counseling is vital to this process; the recovering addict needs to be able to speak with other people who understand what he or she is going through so as not to relapse. In the case of opioid drugs, the recovering addict may take medicine that prevents him or her from getting high from the drugs. Support groups such as Narcotics Anonymous and Alcoholics Anonymous (many drug addicts also have alcohol problems) provide great help for people in recovery.

Overcoming addiction is a lifelong struggle for the person who has a drug problem. Many falter along the way and have

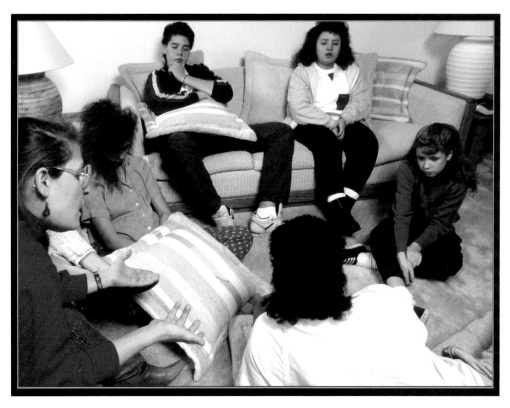

Even after the physical dependence on the drug has ended, the recovering addict needs to break the psychological hold the drug has had on his or her life. Support groups composed of other former addicts can help keep a person from returning to prescription drug abuse.

to repeat the process several times. But with a sincere desire to get clean, and the support of medical personnel and other recovering addicts, it is possible to kick the habit and live a normal life again. However, a recovering addict will always have to stay aware to avoid a relapse.

CHAPTER 4

Prescription Drugs and the Legal System

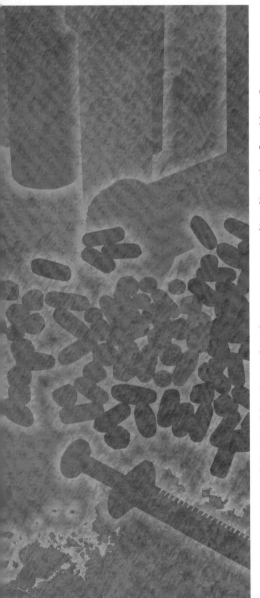

Because prescription drugs can be addictive, they are carefully regulated by the federal government. Only doctors who have had the proper medical training needed to administer drugs can legally prescribe them. Even then, the government puts limits on the amount that can be given to a person over a given period of time.

LEGAL LIMITS

The most powerful painkillers, opioids, belong in a legal category called Schedule II drugs. These drugs have the highest potential for abuse and can be quite addictive. Only doctors with a permit from the U.S. Drug Enforcement Administration (DEA) are allowed to prescribe them. The supply of

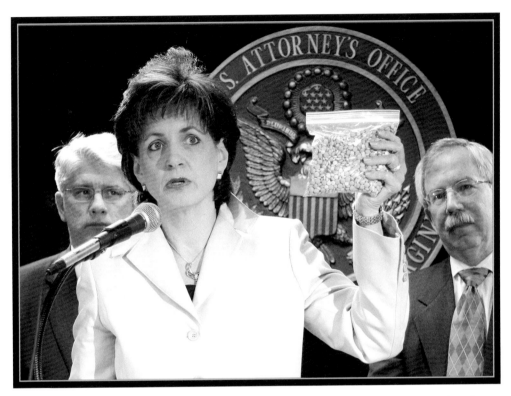

Karen Tandy, head of the U.S. Drug Enforcement Administration, displays a bag of painkillers prescribed by a doctor who was later convicted of illegal drug distribution. This bag was a single day's dose for one patient— an overprescription almost certain to cause abuse or be sold on the black market.

drugs is also tracked by the federal government to make sure they are not stolen or sold on the streets. (The use or sale of prescription drugs as street drugs is called diversion.) Most stimulants also belong to this class, including amphetamines and Ritalin.

Benzodiazepines are Schedule IV drugs and are not as strictly regulated. Patients should be careful when taking these drugs, especially given the dangers of withdrawal from them—fatal

CATEGORIES OF CONTROLLED SUBSTANCES

The Comprehensive Drug Abuse and Prevention Act of 1970 created the current division of drugs sold in America into five schedules, or classes. They're organized by their medical use and potential for misuse. The five schedules are:

Schedule I: These drugs are highly addictive and potentially dangerous; they have no legitimate medical use. They include: heroin, LSD, marijuana, ecstasy (MDMA), mescaline, peyote, PCP, and quaaludes.

Schedule II: These drugs have a high potential for abuse. Prescriptions for them must be given in ink or be typewritten, and they must be signed by the doctor recommending them. No refills are permitted. They include: amphetamine, cocaine, codeine, Dilaudid (hydromorphone), oxycodone (OxyContin, Percodan, Percocet), methamphetamine, methadone, phenobarbital, and Seconal.

Schedule III: These drugs have a potential for abuse. Up to five refills are permitted within six months. They include: anabolic steroids, codeine in low doses mixed with other drugs, hydrocodone mixed with other drugs (Vicodin, Lorcet), and testosterone.

Schedule IV: Some potential for abuse. Up to five refills are permitted in six months. This category includes: alprazolam (Xanax), clonzaepam (Klonopin), lorazepam (Ativan), pentazocine (Talwin), and triazolam (Halcion).

Schedule V: These drugs are only subject to state and local regulation. The potential for abuse is low, and any addictive components are usually mixed with non-addictive drugs. A prescription is not always required. These drugs include: codeine in very low doses mixed with non-addictive drugs (Actifed, Robitussin AC) and buprenorphine (Buprenex).

seizures have been known to occur. In truth, any drug on federal schedules is dangerous and must be used with caution.

PENALTIES FOR DOCTORS AND PHARMACISTS

Doctors who misprescribe drugs face stiff penalties. They may lose their DEA license, or even their medical license, and be unable to work as physicians. Also, they may face criminal charges and have to serve time in jail. Depending on what they have done, these doctors may face both federal and state prosecution. Finally, if people died because of drugs obtained improperly, the prescribing physicians may even be charged with murder. Even if they avoid criminal charges, they may be sued.

Pharmacists face similar penalties for filling illegal prescriptions, or for illegally selling drugs without a prescription. They are also licensed and regulated by the DEA, and the amount of drugs they dispense is monitored and recorded.

MONITORING PRESCRIPTION DRUG USE

In recent years, many states have begun extensive programs to track the usage of prescription drugs. These programs seek to cut down on the abuse of drugs by identifying people who are addicted to them. They also hope to find doctors who are misprescribing the drugs and pharmacists who are illegally dispensing them.

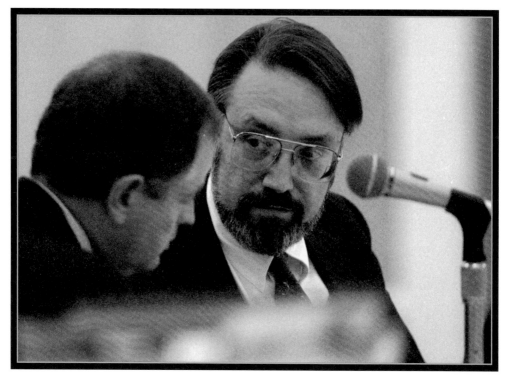

Dr. William Hurwitz was convicted in 2005 for improper drug distribution. He had supplied many prescription drug abusers with massive doses of painkillers, including morphine and OxyContin. He was also convicted for causing the death of a woman who had died of a morphine overdose.

A major tool that is used in these monitoring programs is electronic data transfer (EDT) systems. They immediately transmit information about a prescription to a central database. This allows government officials to easily track data such as the amount of drugs prescribed by a doctor or the number of prescriptions a patient has had filled.

Monitoring programs have been mostly successful in combating prescription drug abuse. For example, in the first five years of

Oklahoma's Schedule II monitoring program, the amount of prescription drugs that undercover agents were able to purchase from drug dealers dropped 61 percent. Since 1972, New York state has used a monitoring plan called the serialized prescription program. Under this program, special forms are used to prescribe drugs, and copies of these forms are kept by the state. In 1989, New York began to track benzodiazepines through this program. Within a year, emergency room admissions for benzodiazepine-related ailments dropped 31 percent.

Drug monitoring programs have their critics. Some have said these programs keep doctors from prescribing drugs to patients who could use them because the doctors don't want the hassle of extra paperwork or don't want to be scrutinized by state regulators. This issue especially comes up with painkillers, which many health-care providers underprescribe out of fear of causing addiction, according to the National Institute of Drug Abuse.

There is probably some truth to these criticisms. Yet when New York state reviewed the results of placing benzodiazepine in its serialized prescription program, it found that the total number of prescriptions had fallen by only 10 percent. It seems that by adding another layer of monitoring, the state had managed to cut down on illegal use of the drug without impacting its proper prescription. It is telling to note that the waves of OxyContin abuse that occurred during the late 1990s and first years of the twenty-first century were most severe in states without any prescription monitoring programs, like Virginia.

Beyond merely tracking the writing of prescriptions, law enforcement officials investigate other activities that allow people to abuse prescription drugs. In large cities, the police may have a special task force or department dedicated to cracking down on prescription drug abuse. Most states have their own investigative departments as well. They concentrate their efforts on three areas: finding doctor-shoppers, finding dealers, and finding health-care workers (doctors and nurses) who are misusing prescription drugs.

Doctor-shoppers, or people who go to many different doctors to get enough of the drug they crave, are usually detected through drug monitoring programs or by doctors or pharmacists they have tried to get drugs from. Many have obvious signs of addiction or make enough visits to attract the suspicion of health-care providers. These people are arrested for violating the laws governing the amount of drugs they are allowed to be prescribed.

Dealers are much rarer than doctor-shoppers. However, arresting a dealer can have a much greater effect than arresting an addict because it dries up the supply. Of course, dealers tend to be doctor-shoppers themselves. They may also steal their supply from hospitals or drugstores. They have been known to forge prescriptions and print their own prescription pads.

It is a sad but true fact that doctors and nurses tend to have higher rates of addiction than the general public does. The stress of their jobs, plus the availability of drugs, can prove to be tragic for many of these health-care providers. Police investigate doctors and nurses they suspect of abusing drugs. Far more dangerous are the doctors who write prescriptions for addicts—they are the target of the doctor-shoppers. Some doctors will get a reputation for writing a prescription for any drug in exchange for their office-visit fee. Little better than pushers themselves, these doctors help to keep addiction alive in many regions.

Finding the appropriate balance between regulating drugs so that their abuse is minimized and giving them to patients who really need them remains a huge challenge for all levels of government and society.

CHAPTER 5
Prescription Drug Abuse and Society

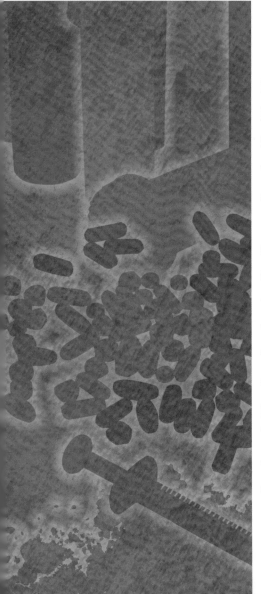

Modern medicine can work miracles. People routinely survive diseases today that would have killed them fifty years ago. Others live without pain, or have richer and fuller lives than they could have had without medication for physical and psychological illnesses.

However, these drugs often have tragic costs. For example, thousands of Civil War soldiers became addicted to morphine, which had spared them the agony of their wounds. Many drugs were considered safe when they were first introduced, only to cause addiction and other potentially fatal problems. Valium, which was said to be "safe as candy," left many people hooked on benzodiazepines, sometimes with deadly results.

Prescription drug abuse is an epidemic that the United States is just becoming aware of. Because the drugs are prescribed by doctors and serve a useful purpose for people with serious conditions, their abuse can take whole communities by surprise. For example, rural regions of the country, like southwestern Virginia and the state of Maine, had never suffered from the kind of drug problems of large cities such as New York or Washington. They were too far away for such illegal drugs as

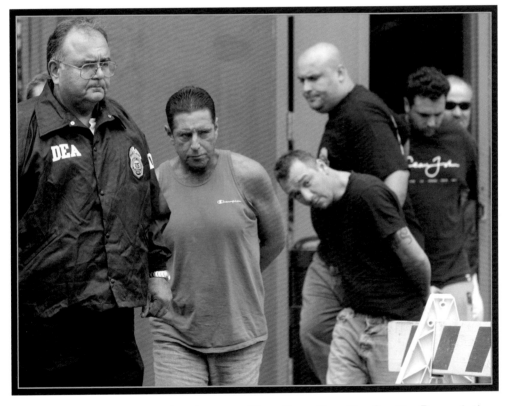

DEA officers arrest people who were illegally selling OxyContin. Prescription drug abuse has caused crime waves in regions that had never before seen drug-related crimes.

heroin or cocaine to have had much of a presence. But after OxyContin was introduced, both of these regions soon had a major crisis on their hands. Drug treatment centers designed to hold ten or fifteen patients a year were swamped with hundreds of recovering addicts. A dangerous and addictive drug had been introduced by doctors in a region where dealers did not go.

Prescription drug abuse affects the entire community in ways that extend far beyond an addict's suffering or the pain it

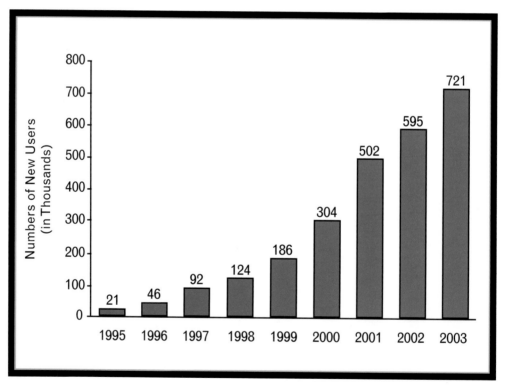

OxyContin was first introduced in 1995 and within eight years had become one of the most frequently prescribed painkillers. This explosion of use led to waves of drug addiction throughout Appalachia, Florida, and other regions of the country.

inflicts on his or her family. Some of the effects are the same as those caused by any drug abuse, but some are peculiar to the abuse of prescription drugs.

One obvious effect is the increase in crime. Like any addict, abusers of prescription drugs need to buy their drugs, and they are not cheap. A single pill can cost twenty or thirty dollars. People who are dependent on prescription drugs often max out their credit cards and deplete their savings accounts to pay for them. When they run out of money, they often turn to crime, stealing things to sell in order to buy more drugs. Thus, a rise in addiction in a region usually brings on a rise in the crime rate. People who are abusing drugs often are not in control of themselves and may become violent, leading to more murders and assaults.

Additionally, prescription drug abuse forces the police to carefully monitor doctors and pharmacies, taking up valuable time that could be spent patrolling neighborhoods or investigating crimes. So, the abuse of these drugs becomes a drain on the entire community.

Prescription drug abuse also impacts the health-care system of a region. First, with the rise in violent crime, there will be more visits to emergency rooms and clinics. Also, addicts tend to neglect their health and get sick more often than they did before becoming dependent. They may also be going through withdrawal and need medical attention.

Also, prescription drug addicts use up time that could be spent treating other patients. By going to the emergency room to get drugs, or faking symptoms while meeting with a doctor, they put a strain on the entire network of services that are needed to support a region's population. Addicts may use up drugs more rapidly than doctors and hospitals expected, causing shortages and denying drugs to people who actually need them.

Another disturbing aspect of prescription drug abuse is that it can go undetected for so long. Many who become hooked started out by getting the drug for a valid medical reason. No one suspects them of abusing the drug, since it's known that they need to take it. Even people who weren't prescribed the drug—such as teenagers who abuse painkillers, tranquilizers, or stimulants—may go unnoticed for a long time because they are taking "medicine." It doesn't help that many people don't realize how serious the abuse of drugs such as Xanax can be—since they are prescribed by doctors, they seem somehow "safe."

The availability of prescription drugs greatly contributes to all of these problems. According to a 2005 study by the National Center on Addiction and Substance Abuse (CASA), many doctors are not well-informed about how to recognize the warning signs of addiction in their patients, or they do not have enough of a patient's medical history to realize that he or she is at a greater-than-normal risk of becoming addicted. Doctors may also not realize that the drugs they are prescribing are dangerously addictive. This was the case with Valium in the 1960s and, more recently, OxyContin.

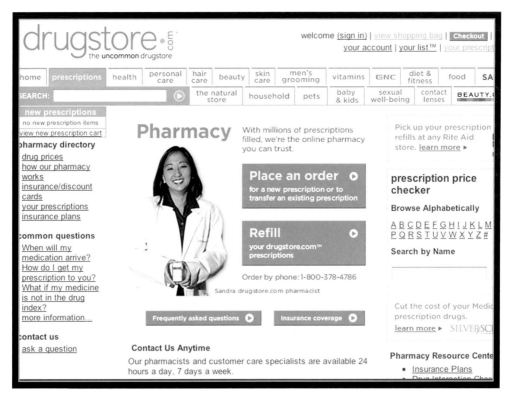

This is the home page of Drugstore.com, an online pharmacy. The Internet has made it easy to order prescription drugs. This has been very helpful to many people with chronic conditions, but unfortunately it has helped many prescription drug addicts to easily get the drugs they are addicted to.

The Internet has helped to make prescription drugs more accessible. Unlike illicit street drugs, like heroin or crack, abusers of prescription drugs don't always have to visit drug dealers to get their fix. Often, they can order them from the privacy of their own home, using a credit card to pay for them. Many sites do not require a prescription in order to complete a sale.

CHAPTER 6

Prescription Drug Abuse and the Media

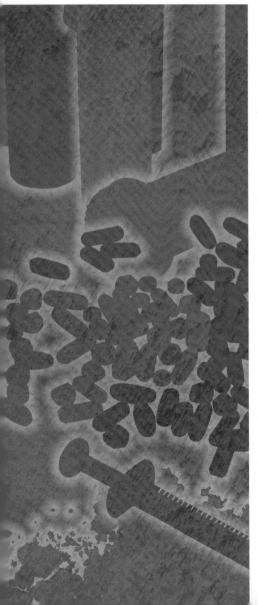

Mathew Perry, Marilyn Monroe, Rush Limbaugh, Chevy Chase, Brett Butler, Jerry Lewis, Judy Garland, Liza Minelli, and Ozzy Osbourne: What do all these celebrities have in common? All have abused prescription drugs at some point in their lives. They are not alone. Thousands of others, famous and unknown, could be listed as well.

AN INVISIBLE EPIDEMIC

Nevertheless, prescription drug abuse doesn't get the same attention as illegal drug abuse does. Robert Downey Jr.'s struggles with heroin and cocaine have made headlines. However, the struggles of fellow actors like Chevy Chase or Mathew Perry—who were hooked on powerful

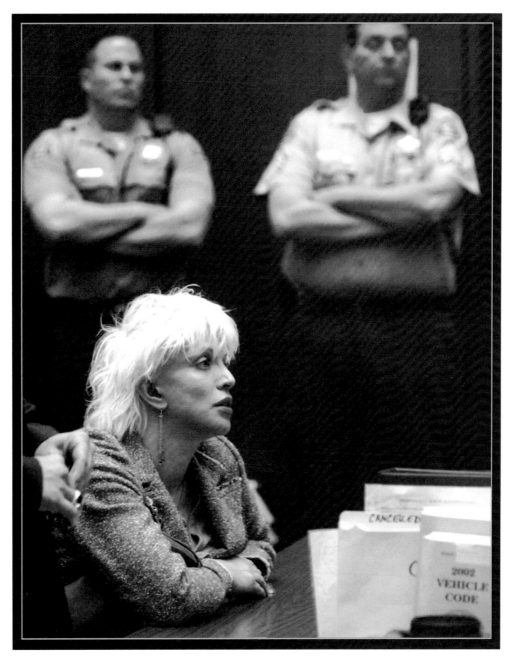

Rock star Courtney Love was sentenced to spend time in a rehabilitation program in 2004 after pleading guilty to illegally using prescription painkillers. The troubled singer has been battling her abuse of prescription drugs for several years. She later violated her probation and was forced to spend six months in rehab in 2005.

opioid painkillers that are as addictive as heroin—barely registered. This neglect by the media and the public has contributed to a creeping epidemic that now threatens almost all of America.

According to CASA, about 7.8 million Americans admitted to having abused prescription drugs in 1992. By 2003, that number almost doubled to 15.1 million. Teens were especially at risk: 2.3 million young people between the ages of twelve and seventeen admitted to abusing prescription drugs, with girls more likely to have an addiction than boys.

Only gradually has the media responded to this explosion in prescription drug abuse. The recent high-profile cases of Rush Limbaugh and Ozzy Osbourne, who both abused prescription painkillers, have helped create awareness among the general public of how addictive these drugs can be and how dangerous they can be when abused. The widespread OxyContin abuse in areas that had never before had large-scale addiction problems also shows just how devastating prescription drug abuse can be.

It is not just painkillers that have come under scrutiny. Ritalin, the stimulant used to treat ADHD, has come under attack in recent years. Many concerned parents have begun to question the diagnosis of ADHD in their children. Some wonder if the syndrome even exists, or, if it does, how common it really is. Many doctors and children's advocates have also criticized the use of such a powerful stimulant as Ritalin in treating young children. Despite the claims of pharmaceutical manufacturers,

Ritalin can be lethal if taken in large quantities. Of course, it is as addictive as any stimulant. Another problem is that some teens who have been prescribed Ritalin sell it to people who are just looking for a buzz or energy boost. This unmonitored use can lead to addiction.

Xanax, the prescription form of benzodiazepine, has come under fire as well. Like Valium before it, Xanax has been marketed as an extremely safe and commonly prescribed remedy for all sorts of complaints, notably anxiety, nervousness, and insomnia. However, like Valium, Xanax can be very addictive. Its overprescription has made it readily available on the street, where it is sometimes used to help people come down from a stimulant or opiate high.

A GENERAL LACK OF AWARENESS

Many drug-abuse prevention advocates believe the media should pay more attention to the problem of prescription drug abuse. A greater media focus will increase awareness of the issues of addiction not only among patients, but among doctors as well. A 2003 study by the National Center for Addiction and Substance Abuse at Columbia University found that more than 40 percent of doctors do not routinely ask patients if they have had past drug abuse problems before they prescribe powerful drugs. More than 30 percent do not routinely call a patient's previous doctors to verify his or her medical history.

On the other hand, the study found that more than 90 percent of doctors had not prescribed drugs out of fear that the patient would become addicted to them. Therefore, many patients who could have benefited from these drugs did not receive them. Had doctors been more vigilant about following up on a patient's history, maybe they would have been more confident about prescribing drugs.

However, care must still be taken in this area. In the 1990s, many stories appeared in the media about how painkillers were underprescribed and that the threat of addiction was greatly exaggerated. Certainly, many people with chronic suffering could benefit from painkillers (and in these extreme cases, the likelihood of addiction is indeed low). Also, it does not make sense to deny terminally ill cancer patients consistent doses of painkillers that would keep them from having the rapid swings between agony and drug-induced stupor that many now have to live through. But as admirable as the goals of the pain-treatment movement were, many people believe that the pendulum has swung too far in this case, contributing greatly to the overprescription (and widespread abuse) of powerful drugs like OxyContin.

CONCLUSION

We live in a time of great advances in medicine. Problems that were untreatable as little as ten years ago can be treated today and even cured—thanks in many cases to the amazing new drugs

Ten Facts About Prescription Drugs

- Prescription drug abuse now affects more than fifteen million Americans. This is greater than the number of people who are addicted to heroin or cocaine.
- Teens are one of the fastest-growing segments of the population to abuse prescription drugs. The number of teens who abuse these drugs has tripled in the last ten years. The number of teens addicted to prescription opiates has shot up 542 percent over that same time period.
- Just because a drug has been prescribed by a doctor does not mean that it is safe or that a person cannot become addicted to it.
- People who are depressed, overweight, under stress, or have a history of alcohol abuse are most at risk of becoming addicted to drugs. Doctors must be very careful in recommending the right drug to them.
- The most common types of prescription drugs people become addicted to are opioid painkillers (Vicodin, Demerol), central nervous system depressants (benzodiazepams, like Xanax), and stimulants (amphetamines, Ritalin).
- More than half a million people die every year as a result of prescription drug abuse.
- Abusing prescription drugs can lower your life expectancy by as much as fifteen years.
- Treatment of prescription drug abuse is complicated by withdrawal symptoms, which are very painful for the patient to go through.
- Recovering addicts will struggle against their addiction for the rest of their lives, but recovery is possible.
- Groups like Narcotics Anonymous and Alcoholics Anonymous can help recovering addicts put their lives back together.

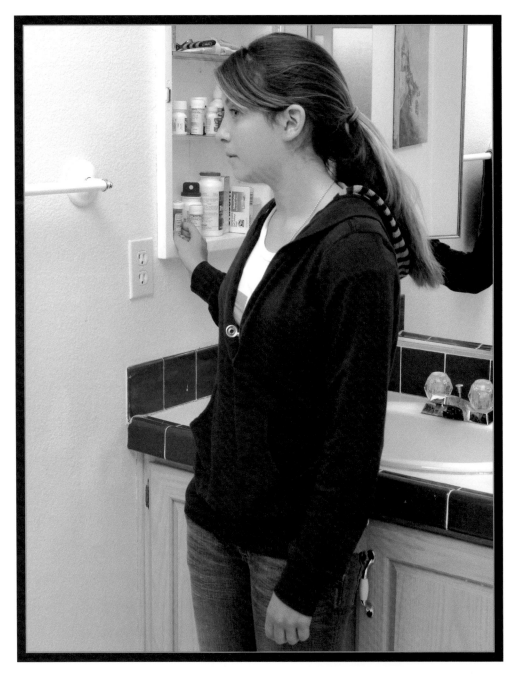

Prescription drugs have the power to cure many problems and help us feel better. But like any power, they must be used responsibly. The choices you make in how you take these drugs are crucial to whether you, or the drugs, will control your life.

that have been created by scientists. For example, HIV infection as little as fifteen years ago was a virtual death sentence. Today, thousands of people live with HIV and never develop AIDS because of the powerful antiviral drugs they take.

However, nearly anything can be abused, and drugs are no different. Some consumer health advocates charge that, in the drive to grow profits, the drug industry has sometimes been too lax in putting drugs that have a high potential for abuse on the market and quick in having doctors prescribe them for more problems than necessary. Doctors, too, have not educated themselves adequately about prescription drug addiction. Most importantly, the public needs to understand that drugs, even when they come from a doctor, can both help and hurt. No drug is completely safe, and it is just as easy to become addicted to a drug from a pharmacy as it is to become addicted to a drug from a dealer. Only an educated medical community—doctors, drug makers, and patients—can hope to reduce the dangers of prescription drug addiction that threaten communities across the United States.

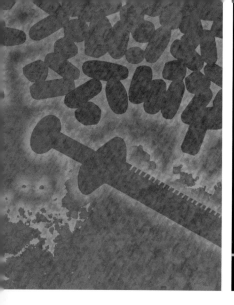

GLOSSARY

abuse The use of a drug for non-medically prescribed reasons.

addiction A physical and emotional dependence on a drug.

benzodiazepine A central nervous system tranquilizer.

circumvent To get around rules and regulations by craftily using weaknesses in a system; to break rules in a clever or crafty way; to evade.

cocaine A powerful illegal stimulant that produces feelings of euphoria.

codeine An opioid painkiller that is often prescribed for post-operative pain.

debilitating Weakening; marked by a pronounced decline in strength and vitality.

Demerol An opioid painkiller that is often used as an anesthetic.

dependency Addiction; the physical need for a drug.

detox Short for detoxification, which is the process of completely ridding the body of a drug.

dispense To prepare and distribute medicine as prescribed.

diversion The illegal sale of prescription drugs.

ecstasy (MDMA) An illegal drug used for the feeling of pleasure and euphoria it creates.

general anaesthesia A state of medically induced complete unconsciousness.

GHB Short for gamma hydroxybutyrate, which is a CNS depressant that causes disorientation.

half-life The time it takes for half of the amount of a drug taken to stop working or be removed from the body.

heroin An illegal opioid that is highly addictive.

illicit Illegal.

marijuana The dried leaves of the cannabis plant, which are illegal.

morphine A powerful opioid painkiller that is highly addictive.

narcotic Any drug that can end pain and is addictive, especially the opioid variety.

opioid A drug that is derived from the opium poppy. Opioids include heroin, morphine, and oxycodone.

oxycodone An opioid painkiller that has the potential to be very addictive.

painkiller Any drug that reduces the sensation of pain.

prescription drug Any drug prescribed by a doctor or that requires a doctor's prescription.

psychological Mental or emotional; having to do with the mind or the processes of the mind.

relapse The recurrence of signs and symptoms of a medical disorder after a period of improvement.

Ritalin A stimulant drug that is used to treat attention deficit hyperactivity disorder, or ADHD.

stimulant Any drug that increases metabolism and energy level.

tolerance The way the body will become used to a drug and need more and more of it to have the desired effect.

tranquilizer A drug that depresses the central nervous system, making users more calm and drowsy.

Valium An early benzodiazepine that is used to treat nervousness or insomnia.

withdrawal The experience a drug user goes through when he or she stops taking a drug, due to the person's dependence on it. Withdrawal symptoms usually include chills, tremors, vomiting, and insomnia.

Xanax A commonly prescribed benzodiazepine that is used to treat anxiety.

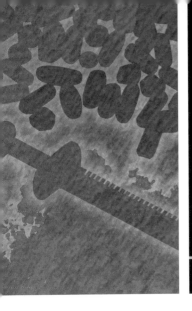

FOR MORE INFORMATION

Addiction Resource Guide
P.O. Box 8612
Tarrytown, NY 10591
(914) 725-5151
Web site: http://www.
 addictionresourceguide.com

Alcoholics Anonymous
P.O. Box 459
New York, NY 10163
(212) 870-3400
Web site: http://www.
 alcoholics-anonymous.org

Nar-Anon Family Group
 Headquarters
22527 Crenshaw Blvd,
 Suite 200B

Torrance, CA 90505
Web site: http://
 www.naranonmi.org/
 meetings_worldwide

Narcotics Anonymous
P.O. Box 9999
Van Nuys, CA 91409
(818) 773-9999
Web site: http://
 www.na.org

Prescription Anonymous, Inc.
P.O. Box 10534
Gathersburg, MD
 20898-0534
Web site: http://www.
 prescriptionanonymous.org

WEB SITES

Due to the changing nature of Internet links, the Rosen Publishing Group, Inc., has developed an online list of Web sites related to the subject of this book. This site is updated regularly. Please use this link to access the list:

http://www.rosenlinks.com/ das/pres

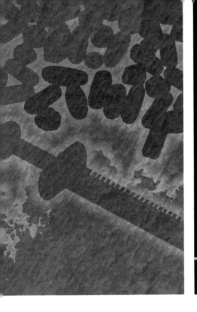

FOR FURTHER READING

Bernards, Neal, ed. *War on Drugs.* San Diego, CA: Greenhaven Press, Inc. 1990.

Colvin, Rod. *Prescription Drug Addiction: The Hidden Epidemic.* Omaha, NE: Addicus Books, 2002.

Gadsby, Joan E. *Addiction By Prescription.* Toronto, ON: Key Porter Books, 2000.

Greenfield, Daniel. *Prescription Drug Abuse and Dependence.* Springfield, IL: Charles C. Thomas Publisher Ltd., 1994.

Grilly, David M. *Drugs and Human Behavior.* Boston, MA: Allyn & Bacon, 2006.

Kuhn, Cynthia, et at. *Buzzed: The Straight Facts About the Most Used and Abused Drugs from Alcohol to Ecstacy.* New York, NY: W. W. Norton, 2003.

Mogil, Cindy R. *Swallowing a Bitter Pill.* New York, NY: New Horizons Press, 2001.

Olive, M. Foster. *Prescription Pain Relievers* (Drugs: the Straight Facts). Philadelphia, PA: Chelsea House Publications, 2005.

Pinsky, Drew. *When Painkillers Become Dangerous: What Everyone Needs to Know About OxyContin and Other Prescription Drugs.* Center City: Hazelden, 2004.

Sora, Joseph, ed. *Substance Abuse.* New York, NY: The H.W. Wilson Company, 1997.

Watkins, Christine, ed. *Prescription Drugs.* San Diego, CA: Greenhaven Press, Inc., 2006.

Wekesser, Carol, ed. *Chemical Dependency: Opposing Viewpoints.* San Diego, CA: Greenhaven Press, Inc., 1997.

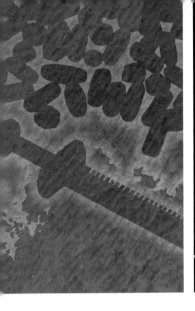

BIBLIOGRAPHY

Colvin, Rob. *Prescription Drug Addiction.* Omaha, NE: Addicus Books, 2002.

Meier, Barry. *Pain Killer.* New York, NY: Rodale Books, 2003.

Breggin, Peter R. *Talking Back to Ritalin.* Monroe, ME: Common Courage Press, 1998.

"Prescription Drugs: Abuse and Addiction" U.S. Department of Health and Human Services, 2005. Retrieved January 2006 (http://www.nida.nih.gov/ResearchReports/Prescription/Prescription.html).

"15 Million in U.S. Abusing Prescription Drugs" *Reuters News Service*, July 11, 2005. Retrieved January 2006 (http://msnbc.msn.com/id/8498679/).

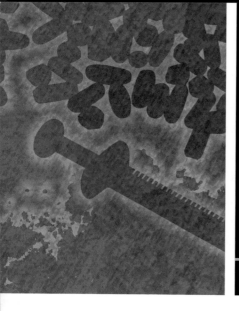

INDEX

A

Alcoholics Anonymous (AA), 30, 51
amphetamine, 33, 34, 51
attention deficit hyperactivity disorder (ADHD), 15, 48

B

barbiturate, 12, 51
benzodiazepine, 12, 18, 29, 30, 33, 37, 40, 49, 51

C

central nervous system (CNS) depressant, 12, 15, 51
cocaine, 4, 6, 10, 34, 42, 46, 51
codeine, 6, 34
Comprehensive Drug Abuse and Prevention Act of 1970, 34

D

Demerol, 6, 10, 24, 51
dependence, 11, 28, 29, 30, 43

detoxification, 29, 30
doctor-shopping, 20, 38, 39
Drug Enforcement Administration (DEA), 32, 35

E

ecstasy (MDMA), 4, 34
electronic date transfer (EDT), 36

G

gamma hydroxybutyrate (GHB), 6

H

Halcion, 12, 34
half-lives, 29
heroin, 4, 10, 34, 42, 45, 46, 48, 51

I

Internet, 45

L

LSD, 34

M

marijuana, 4, 34
methamphetamine, 15
monitoring program, 20-21, 35-37, 38
morphine, 10, 40

N

Narcotics Anonymous (NA), 27, 30, 51
National Center for Addiction and
  Substance Abuse (NCASA), 49
National Institute on Drug Abuse
  (NIDA), 5

O

opioid, 9, 10, 11, 23, 30, 32, 48, 51
over the counter (OTC), 5, 13
OxyContin, 10, 34, 37, 42, 44, 48, 50

P

painkiller, 5, 8, 9, 10, 13, 23, 24, 32,
  37, 44, 48, 50, 51
Percocet, 24, 34
prescription drugs
  abuse among teenagers, 5–6, 19,
    23–27, 44, 48, 51
  acquisition of, 5, 6, 8, 10, 18-19, 20,
    24, 26, 38, 39, 45
  categories of, 8, 34, 51
  celebrity abuse of, 46, 48
  effects of abuse, 6, 11, 12-13, 15, 16,
    19, 22, 24, 27, 29, 30, 33, 35, 40,
    41, 42-43, 51
  legal consequences of abuse, 7, 27,
    29, 35, 38, 43
  media portrayal of, 7, 46, 48, 49, 50
  myths and facts about, 13, 15
  warning signs of addiction to,
    17–19, 27–28, 38, 44, 51

Q

quaaludes, 34

R

relapse, 31
Ritalin, 5, 6, 15, 16, 33, 48–49, 51

S

serialized prescription program, 37
stimulant, 5, 6, 8, 13, 15, 16, 44, 48,
  49, 51

T

tolerance, 11, 19
tranquilizer, 8, 12, 19, 44

V

Valium, 12, 40, 44, 49
Vicodin, 10, 23, 24, 34, 51

X

Xanax, 6, 12, 34, 44, 49, 51

ABOUT THE AUTHOR

Fred Ramen has written several books on diseases and health for the Rosen Publishing Group, including books on tuberculosis and SARS. He was recently a participant in the *Jeopardy! Ultimate Tournament of Champions*. Ramen lives in New York City.

PHOTO CREDITS

P. 5 © Burger/Phanie/Photo Researchers, Inc.; p. 9 © Pallava Bagla/Corbis; p. 11 © Kairos, Latin Stock/Photo Researchers, Inc. p. 14 ©AJPhoto/Photo Researchers, Inc.; p. 18 © John Powell/Peter Arnold, Inc.; p. 21 © Michael A. Keller/zefa/ Corbis; p. 22 © John Cole/Photo Researchers; p. 25 © Keith/ Custom Medical Stock Photo; p. 31 © Beebe/Custom Medical Stock Photo; p. 33 © AP/Wide World Photos; p. 36 Stuart T. Wagner/Richmond Times; p 41 © Tony Kurdzuk/Star Ledger/ Corbis; p, 42 Provided by Substance Abuse and Mental Health Services Administration (SAMHSA); p. 47 © Getty Images; p. 52 © Felicia Martinez/PhotoEdit.

Designer: Tahara Anderson; Editor: Wayne Anderson
Photo Researcher: Marty Levick

9/2007

615
RAM

Ramen, Fred.

Pr 615
RAM   Ramen, Fred.

Prescription
drugs.

$29.25   3731800030848

DATE	BORROWER'S NAME	

BAKER & TAYLOR